The Ultimate Air Fryer Dessert Cooking Guide

Delicious Air Fryer Dessert Recipes For Everyone

Ellie Sloan

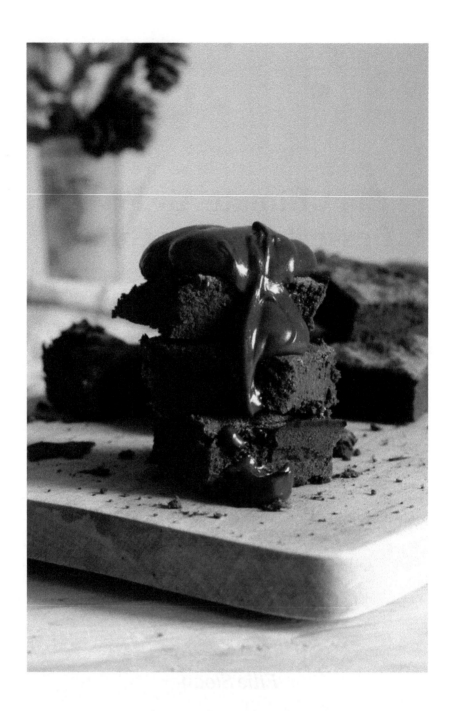

Table of contents

Easy Pears Dessert

Preparation Time: 10 minutes

Cooking Time: 25 minutes

Servings: 12

Ingredients:

- 6 big pears, cored and chopped
- ½ cup raisins
- 1 tsp. ginger powder
- ¼ cup coconut sugar
- 1 tsp. lemon zest, grated

Directions:

1. In a container that fits your Air Fryer, mix pears with raisins, ginger, sugar and lemon zest, stir, introduce in the fryer and cook at 350°F for 25 minutes.
2. Divide into bowls and serve cold.

Nutrition:

Calories 200

Fat 3g

Carbs 6g

Protein 6g

Vanilla Strawberry Mix

Preparation Time: 10 minutes

Cooking Time: 20 minutes

Servings: 10

Ingredients:

- 2 tbsp. lemon juice
- 2 lb. strawberries
- 4 cups coconut sugar
- 1 tsp. cinnamon powder
- 1 tsp. vanilla extract

Directions:

1. In a pot that fits your Air Fryer, mix strawberries with coconut sugar, lemon juice, cinnamon and vanilla, stir gently, introduce in the fryer and cook at 350°F for 20 minutes
2. Divide into bowls and serve cold.

Nutrition:

Calories 140

Fat 0g

Carbs 5g

Protein 2g

Sweet Bananas and Sauce

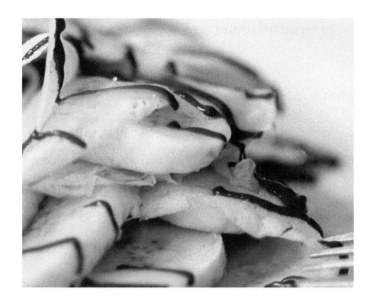

Preparation Time: 10 minutes

Cooking Time: 20 minutes

Servings: 4

Ingredients:

- Juice of ½ lemon
- 3 tbsp. agave nectar

- 1 tbsp. coconut oil
- 4 bananas, peeled and sliced diagonally
- ½ tsp. cardamom seeds

Directions:

1. Arrange bananas in a pan that fits your Air Fryer, add agave nectar, lemon juice, oil and cardamom, introduce in the fryer and cook at 360°F for 20 minutes
2. Divide bananas and sauce between plates and serve.

Nutrition:

Calories 210

Fat 1g

Carbs 8g

Protein 3g

Cinnamon Apples and Mandarin Sauce

Preparation Time: 10 minutes

Cooking Time: 20 minutes

Servings: 4

Ingredients:

- 4 apples, cored, peeled and cored
- 2 cups mandarin juice
- ¼ cup maple syrup
- 2 tsp.s cinnamon powder
- 1 tbsp. ginger, grated

Directions:

1. In a pot that fits your Air Fryer, mix apples with mandarin juice, maple syrup, cinnamon and ginger, introduce in the fryer and cook at 365°F for 20 minutes
2. Divide apples mix between plates and serve warm.

Nutrition:

Calories 170

Fat 1g

Carbs 6g

Protein 4g

Chocolate Vanilla Bars

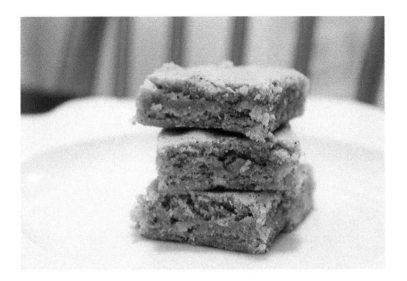

Preparation Time: 10 minutes

Cooking Time: 7 minutes

Servings: 12

Ingredients:

- 1 cup sugar free and vegan chocolate chips
- 2 tbsp. coconut butter
- 2/3 cup coconut cream

- 2 tbsp. stevia
- ¼ tsp. vanilla extract

Directions:

1. Put the cream in a bowl, add stevia, butter and chocolate chips and stir
2. Leave aside for 5 minutes, stir well and mix the vanilla.
3. Transfer the mix into a lined baking sheet, introduce in your Air Fryer and cook at 356°F for 7 minutes.
4. Leave the mix aside to cool down, slice and serve.

Nutrition:

Calories 120

Fat 5g

Carbs 6g

Protein 1g

Raspberry Bars

Preparation Time: 10 minutes

Cooking Time: 6 minutes

Servings: 12

Ingredients:

- ½ cup coconut butter, melted
- ½ cup coconut oil
- ½ cup raspberries, dried
- ¼ cup swerve
- ½ cup coconut, shredded

Directions:

1. In your food processor, blend dried berries very well.
2. In a bowl that fits your Air Fryer, mix oil with butter, swerve, coconut and raspberries, toss well, introduce in the fryer and cook at 320°F for 6 minutes.
3. Spread this on a lined baking sheet, keep in the fridge for an hour, slice and serve.

Nutrition:

Calories 164

Fat 22g

Carbs 4g

Protein 2g

Cocoa Berries Cream

Preparation Time: 10 minutes

Cooking Time: 10 minutes

Servings: 4

Ingredients:

- 3 tbsp. cocoa powder
- 14 oz. coconut cream
- 1 cup blackberries
- 1 cup raspberries
- 2 tbsp. stevia

Directions:

1. In a bowl, whisk cocoa powder with stevia and cream and stir.
2. Add raspberries and blackberries, toss gently, transfer to a pan that fits your Air Fryer, introduce in the fryer and cook at 350°F for 10 minutes.
3. Divide into bowls and serve cold.

Nutrition:

Calories 205

Fat 34g

Carbs 6g

Protein 2g

Cocoa Pudding

Preparation Time: 10 minutes

Cooking Time: 20 minutes

Servings: 2

Ingredients:

- 2 tbsp. water
- ½ tbsp. agar
- 4 tbsp. stevia
- 4 tbsp. cocoa powder
- 2 cups coconut milk, hot

Directions:

1. In a bowl, mix milk with stevia and cocoa powder and stir well.
2. In a bowl, mix agar with water, stir well, add to the cocoa mix, stir and transfer to a pudding pan that fits your Air Fryer.

3. Introduce in the fryer and cook at 356°F for 20 minutes.
4. Serve the pudding cold.

Nutrition:

Calories 170

Fat 2g

Carbs 4g

Protein 3g

Blueberry Coconut Crackers

Preparation Time: 10 minutes

Cooking Time: 30 minutes

Servings: 12

Ingredients:

- ½ cup coconut butter
- ½ cup coconut oil, melted
- 1 cup blueberries
- 3 tbsp. coconut sugar

Directions:

1. In a pot that fits your Air Fryer, mix coconut butter with coconut oil, raspberries and sugar, toss, introduce in the fryer and cook at 367°F for 30 minutes
2. Spread on a lined baking sheet, keep in the fridge for a few hours, slice crackers and serve.

Nutrition:

Calories 174

Fat 5g

Carbs 4g

Protein 7g

Cauliflower Pudding

Preparation Time: 10 minutes

Cooking Time: 30 minutes

Servings: 4

Ingredients:

- 2½ cups water
- 1 cup coconut sugar
- 2 cups cauliflower rice
- 2 cinnamon sticks
- ½ cup coconut, shredded

Directions:

1. In a pot that fits your Air Fryer, mix water with coconut sugar, cauliflower rice, cinnamon and coconut, stir, introduce in the fryer and cook at 365°F for 30 minutes
2. Divide pudding into cups and serve cold.

Nutrition:

Calories 203

Fat 4g

Carbs 9g

Protein 4g

Sweet Vanilla Rhubarb

Preparation Time: 10 minutes

Cooking Time: 10 minutes

Servings: 4

Ingredients:

- 5 cups rhubarb, chopped
- 2 tbsp. coconut butter, melted
- 1/3 cup water
- 1 tbsp. stevia
- 1 tsp. vanilla extract

Directions:

1. Put rhubarb, ghee, water, stevia and vanilla extract in a pan that fits your Air Fryer, introduce in the fryer and cook at 365°F for 10 minutes
2. Divide into small bowls and serve cold.

Nutrition:

Calories 103

Fat 2g

Carbs 6g

Protein 2g

Shortbread fingers

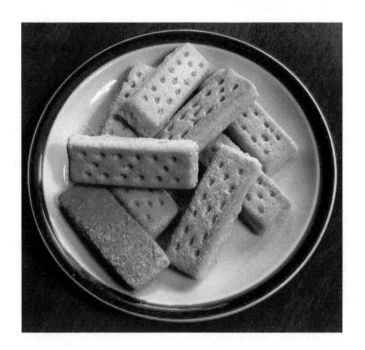

Preparation Time: 10 minutes

Cooking time: 12 minutes

Serving: 12

Ingredients:

- 6 oz. Butter

- 2.6 oz. Caster sugar
- 9 oz. Plain flour

Directions:

1. Mix flour with sugar and butter in a bowl.
2. Knead this shortbread dough well until smooth.
3. Make 4-finger shapes out of this dough and place them in the Air Fryer basket.
4. Air fry for 12 minutes at 350°F
5. Flip the shortbread cookies after 6 minutes then resume cooking
6. Serve.

Nutrition:

Calories 204

Fat 12g

Carbs 22.2g

Protein 2.3g

Fruit crumble pie

Preparation Time: 10 minutes

Cooking time: 15 minutes

Serving: 6

Ingredients:

- 6 oz. Plain flour
- 1 oz. Butter
- 1 oz. Caster sugar
- 1 medium red apple, peeled and diced
- medium plums, diced
- 1 oz. Frozen berries, diced
- 1 tsp. cinnamon

Directions:

1. Toss all the fruits into the Air Fryer Basket
2. Whisk flour with sugar and butter to make a crumble
3. Spread this crumble over the fruits evenly

4. Select 15 minutes of cooking time at 350°F, then press "start."
5. Once the Air Fryer beeps, remove the basket
6. Slice and serve.

Nutrition:

Calories 149

Fat 4.8g

Carbs 26.3g

Protein 1.9g

Chocolate mug cake

Preparation Time: 7 minutes

Cooking time: 13 minutes

Serving: 3

Ingredients:

- ½ cup of cocoa powder
- ½ cup stevia powder
- 1 cup coconut cream
- 1 package cream cheese, room temperature
- 1 tbsp. Vanilla extract
- 1 tbsp. Butter

Directions:

1. Preheat the Air Fryer for 5 minutes at 350°F.
2. In a mixing bowl, combine all the listed ingredients using a hand mixer until fluffy.
3. Pour into greased mugs.

4. Place the mugs in the fryer basket and bake for 13 minutes at 350°F.
5. Serve when cool.

Nutrition:

Calories 744

Fat 69.7g

Carbs 4g

Protein 13.9g

Fried peaches

Preparation Time: 2 hours 10 minutes

Ccooking time: 15 minutes

Servings: 4

Ingredients:

- 4 Ripe peaches
- 1½ cup flour
- Salt to taste
- 4 egg yolks
- 3/4 cups cold water
- 1 1/2 tbsp. Olive oil
- tbsp. Brandy
- 4 egg whites
- Cinnamon/sugar mix

Directions:

1. Mix flour, egg yolks, and salt in a mixing bowl.
2. Slowly mix in water, then add brandy.

3. Set the mixture aside for 2 hours and meanwhile cut an x at the bottom of each peach.
4. Boil some water and fill a large bowl with water and ice.
5. Boil each peach for about a minute, then plunge them in the ice bath.
6. The peels should fall off the peach.
7. Beat the egg whites and mix into the batter.
8. Dip each peach in the mix to coat. Pour the coated peach into the oven rack/basket.
9. Place the rack on the middle-shelf of the Air Fryer oven.
10. Set temperature to 360°F and set time to 10 minutes.
11. Prepare a plate with cinnamon/sugar mix, roll peaches in the mix and serve.

Nutrition:

Calories 306

Carbs 12g

Protein 10g

Apple dumplings

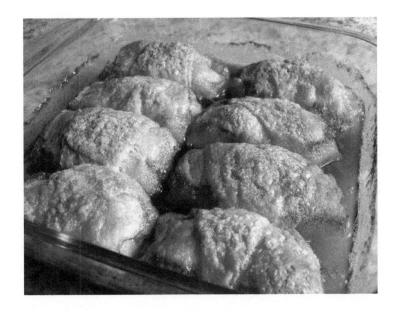

Preparation Time: 7 minutes

Cooking time: 25 minutes

Serving: 4

Ingredients:

- tbsp. Melted coconut oil
- puff pastry sheets

- 1 tbsp. Brown sugar
- tbsp. Raisins
- small apples, peeled and cored

Directions:

1. Preheat your Air Fryer oven to 356°F
2. Mix apples with raisins and sugar
3. Place a bit of apple mixture into puff pastry sheets and brush sides with melted coconut oil.
4. Place into the Air Fryer. Cook 25 minutes, turning halfway through. Remove from the oven when golden.

Nutrition:

Calories 367

Fat 7g

Carbs 5g

Protein 2g

Apple pie

Preparation Time: 5 minutes

Cooking time: 30 minutes

Serving: 4

Ingredients:

- ½ tsp. Vanilla extract
- 1 beaten egg
- 1 large apple, chopped
- 1 pillsbury
- Pie crust
- 1 tbsp. Butter
- 1 tbsp. Ground cinnamon
- 1 tbsp. Raw sugar
- tbsp. Sugar
- tsp. Lemon juice
- Baking spray

Directions:

1. Lightly grease baking pan of Air Fryer oven with cooking spray.
2. Spread the pie crust on the bottom of the pan up to the sides.
3. In a bowl, mix vanilla, sugar, cinnamon, lemon juice, and apples and pour on top of the pie crust.
4. Top apples with butter slices, then cover apples with the other pie crust.
5. Prick the pie's top with a knife.
6. Spread beaten egg on top of crust and sprinkle sugar.
7. For 30 minutes, cook on 350°F
8. Remove when tops are browned.
9. Serve and enjoy.

Nutrition:

Calories 372

Fat 19g

Carbs 5g

Protein 4.2g

Cinnamon Rolls

Preparation Time: 2 hours

Cooking Time: 15 minutes

Servings: 8

Ingredients:

- 1 lb. vegan bread dough
- ¾ cup coconut sugar
- 1 and ½ tbsp. cinnamon powder
- 2 tbsp. vegetable oil

Directions:

1. Roll dough on a floured working surface, shape a rectangle and brush with the oil.
2. In a bowl, mix cinnamon with sugar, stir, sprinkle this over dough, roll into a log, seal well and cut into 8 pieces.

3. Leave rolls to rise for 2 hours, place them in your Air Fryer's basket, cook at 350°F for 5 minutes, flip them, cook for 4 minutes more and transfer to a platter.

Nutrition:

Calories 170

Fat 1g

Carbs 7g

Protein 6g

Cherries and Rhubarb Bowls

Preparation Time: 10 minutes

Cooking Time: 35 minutes

Servings: 4

Ingredients:

- 2 cups cherries, pitted and halved
- 1 cup rhubarb, sliced
- 1 cup apple juice
- 2 tbsp. sugar
- ½ cup raisins.

Directions:

In a pot that fits your Air Fryer, combine the cherries with the rhubarb and the other ingredients, toss, cook at 330°F for 35 minutes, divide into bowls, cool down and serve.

Nutrition:

Calories 212

Fat 8g

Carbs 13g

Protein 7g

Pumpkin Bowls

Preparation Time: 10 minutes

Cooking Time: 15 minutes

Servings: 4

Ingredients:

- 2 cups pumpkin flesh, cubed
- 1 cup heavy cream
- 1 tsp. cinnamon powder
- 3 tbsp. sugar
- 1 tsp. nutmeg, ground

Directions:

1. In a pot that fits your Air Fryer, combine the pumpkin with the cream and the other ingredients, introduce in the fryer and cook at 360°F for 15 minutes.
2. Divide into bowls and serve.

Nutrition:

Calories 212

Fat 5g

Carbs 15g

Protein 7g

Apple Jam

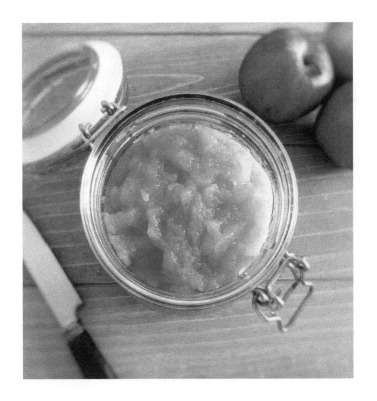

Preparation Time: 10 minutes

Cooking Time: 25 minutes

Servings: 4

Ingredients:

- 1 cup water
- ½ cup sugar
- 1-lb. apples, cored, peeled and chopped
- ½ tsp. nutmeg, ground

Directions:

1. In a pot that suits your Air Fryer, mix the apples with the water and the other ingredients, toss, introduce the pan in the fryer and cook at 370°F for 25 minutes.
2. Blend a bit using an immersion blender, divide into jars and serve.

Nutrition:

Calories 204

Fat 3g

Carbs 12g

Protein 4g

Yogurt and Pumpkin Cream

Preparation Time: 10 minutes

Cooking Time: 30 minutes

Servings: 4

Ingredients:

- 1 cup yogurt
- 1 cup pumpkin puree
- 2 eggs, whisked
- 2 tbsp. sugar
- ½ tsp. vanilla extract

Directions:

1. In a large bowl, mix the puree and the yogurt with the other ingredients, whisk well, pour into 4 ramekins, put them in the Air Fryer and cook at 370°F for 30 minutes.
2. Cool down and serve.

Nutrition:

Calories 192

Fat 7g

Carbs 12g

Protein 4g

Raisins Rice Mix

Preparation Time: 10 minutes

Cooking Time: 25 minutes

Servings: 6

Ingredients:

- 1 cup white rice
- 2cups coconut milk
- 3tbsp. sugar
- 1 tsp. vanilla extract
- ½ cup raisins

Directions:

1. In the Air Fryer's pan, combine the rice with the milk and the other ingredients, introduce the pan in the fryer and cook at 320°F for 25 minutes.
2. Divide into bowls and serve warm.

Nutrition:

Calories 132

Fat 6g

Carbs 11g

Protein 7g

Orange Bowls

Preparation Time: 10 minutes

Cooking Time: 10 minutes

Servings: 4

Ingredients:

- 1 cup oranges, peeled and cut into segments
- 1 cup cherries, pitted and halved
- 1 cup mango, peeled and cubed
- 1 cup orange juice
- 2 tbsp. sugar

Directions:

1. In the Air Fryer's pan, mix the oranges with the cherries and the other ingredients, toss and cook at 320°F for 10 minutes.
2. Divide into bowls and serve cold.

Nutrition:

Calories 191

Fat 7g

Carbs 14g

Protein 4g

Strawberry Jam

Preparation Time: 10 minutes

Cooking Time: 25 minutes

Servings: 8

Ingredients:

- 1 lb. strawberries, chopped
- 1 tbsp. lemon zest, grated
- 1 and ½ cups water
- ½ cup sugar
- ½ tbsp. lemon juice

Directions:

1. In the Air Fryer's pan, mix the berries with the water and the other ingredients, stir, introduce the pan in your Air Fryer and cook at 330°F for 25 minutes.
2. Divide into bowls and serve cold.

Nutrition:

Calories 202

Protein 7g

Fat 8g

Carbs 6g

Caramel Cream

Preparation Time: 10 minutes

Cooking Time: 15 minutes

Servings: 4

Ingredients:

- 1 cup heavy cream
- 3 tbsp. caramel syrup
- ½ cup coconut cream
- 1 tbsp. sugar
- ½ tsp. cinnamon powder

Directions:

1. In a bowl, mix the cream with the caramel syrup and the other ingredients, whisk, divide into small ramekins, introduce in the fryer and cook at 320°F and bake for 15 minutes.
2. Divide into bowls and serve cold.

Nutrition:

Calories 234

Fat 13g

Carbs 11g

Protein 5g

Wrapped Pears

Preparation Time: 10 minutes

Cooking Time: 15 minutes

Servings: 4

Ingredients:

- 4 puff pastry sheets
- 14 oz. vanilla custard
- 2 pears, halved
- 1 egg, whisked
- 2tbsp. sugar

Directions:

1. Put the puff pastry slices on a clean surface, add spoonful of vanilla custard in the center of each, top with pear halves and wrap.
2. Brush pears with egg, sprinkle sugar and place them in your Air Fryer's basket and cook at 320°F for 15 minutes.

3. Divide parcels on plates and serve.

Nutrition:

Calories 200

Fat 7g

Carbs 6g

Protein 6g

Perfect Cinnamon Toast

Preparation Time: 10 minutes

Cooking Time: 5 minutes

Servings: 6

Ingredients:

- 2 tsp. pepper
- 1 ½ tsp. cinnamon
- ½ C. sweetener of choice
- 1 C. coconut oil
- 12 slices whole wheat bread

Directions:

1. Melt coconut oil and mix with sweetener until dissolved. Mix in remaining ingredients minus bread till incorporated.
2. Spread mixture onto bread, covering all area.
3. Pour the coated pieces of bread into the Oven rack/basket. Place the Rack on the middle-shelf of

the Air Fryer oven. Set temperature to 400°F, and set time to 5 minutes.

4. Remove and cut diagonally. Enjoy!

Nutrition:

Calories 124

Fat 2g

Carbs 5g

Protein 0g

Angel Food Cake

Preparation Time: 5 minutes

Cooking Time: 30 minutes

Servings: 12

Ingredients:

- ¼ cup butter, melted
- 1 cup powdered erythritol
- 1 tsp. strawberry extract
- 12 egg whites
- 2 tsp.s cream of tartar

Directions:

1. Preheat the Air Fryer oven for 5 minutes.
2. Blend the cream of tartar and egg whites.
3. Use a hand mixer and whisk until white and fluffy.
4. Add the rest of the ingredients except for the butter and whisk for another minute.
5. Pour into a baking dish.

6. Place in the Air Fryer basket and cook for 30 minutes at 400°F or if a toothpick inserted in the middle comes out clean.
7. Drizzle with melted butter once cooled.

Nutrition:

Calories 65

Fat 5g

Carbs 6.2g

Protein 3.1g

Chocolate Donuts

Preparation Time: 5 minutes

Cooking Time: 20 minutes

Servings: 8-10

Ingredients:

- (8 oz.) can jumbo biscuits
- Cooking oil
- Chocolate sauce, such as Hershey's

Directions:

1. Separate the biscuit dough into 8 biscuits and place them on a flat work surface. Use a small circle cookie cutter or a biscuit cutter to cut a hole in the center of each biscuit. You can also cut the holes using a knife.
2. Grease the basket with cooking oil.
3. Place 4 donuts in the Air Fryer oven. Do not stack. Spray with cooking oil. Cook for 4 minutes at 390°F.

4. Open the Air Fryer and flip the donuts. Cook for an additional 4 minutes.
5. Remove the cooked donuts from the Air Fryer oven, then repeat for the remaining 4 donuts.
6. Drizzle chocolate sauce over the donuts and enjoy while warm.

Nutrition:

Calories 181

Fat 98g

Carbs 42g

Protein 3g

Apple Hand Pies

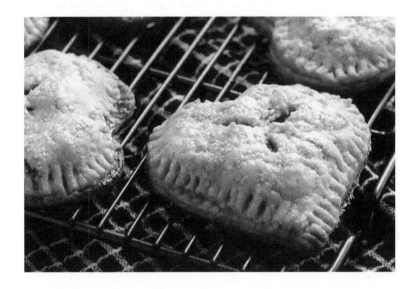

Preparation Time: 5 minutes

Cooking Time: 8 minutes

Servings: 6

Ingredients:

- 15 oz. no-sugar-added apple pie filling
- 1 store-bought crust

Directions:

1. Lay out pie crust and slice into equal-sized squares.
2. Place 2 tbsp. filling into each square and seal crust with a fork.
3. Pour into the Oven rack/basket. Place the Rack on the middle-shelf of the Air Fryer oven. Set temperature to 390°F, and set time to 8 minutes until golden in color.

Nutrition:

Calories 278

Fat 10g

Carbs 17g

Protein 5g

Sweet Cream Cheese Wontons

Preparation Time: 5 minutes

Cooking Time: 5 minutes

Servings: 16

Ingredients:

- 1 egg with a little water
- Wonton wrappers
- ½ C. powdered erythritol
- 8 oz. softened cream cheese
- Olive oil

Directions:

1. Mix sweetener and cream cheese together.
2. Lay out 4 wontons at a time and cover with a dish towel to prevent drying out.
3. Place ½ of a tsp. of cream cheese mixture into each wrapper.

4. Dip finger into egg/water mixture and fold diagonally to form a triangle. Seal edges well.
5. Repeat with remaining ingredients.
6. Place filled wontons into the Air Fryer oven and cook 5 minutes at 400°F, shaking halfway through cooking.

Nutrition:

Calories 303

Fat 3g

Carbs 3g

Protein 0.5g

French Toast Bites

Preparation Time: 5 minutes

Cooking Time: 15 minutes

Servings: 8

Ingredients:

- Almond milk
- Cinnamon
- Sweetener
- 3 eggs
- 4 pieces wheat bread

Directions:

1. Preheat the Air Fryer oven to 360°F.
2. Whisk eggs and thin out with almond milk.
3. Mix 1/3 cup of sweetener with lots of cinnamon.
4. Tear bread in half, ball up pieces and press together to form a ball.

5. Soak bread balls in egg and then roll into cinnamon sugar, making sure to thoroughly coat.
6. Place coated bread balls into the Air Fryer oven and bake 15 minutes.

Nutrition:

Calories 289

Fat 11g

Carbs 17g

Protein 0g

Cinnamon Sugar Roasted Chickpeas

Preparation Time: 5 minutes

Cooking Time: 10 minutes

Servings: 2

Ingredients:

- 1 tbsp. sweetener
- 1 tbsp. cinnamon
- 1 cup chickpeas

Directions:

1. Preheat Air Fryer oven to 390°F.
2. Rinse and drain chickpeas.
3. Mix all ingredients together and add to Air Fryer.
4. Pour into the Oven rack/basket. Place the Rack on the middle-shelf of the Air Fryer oven. Set temperature to 390°F, and set time to 10 minutes.

Nutrition:

Calories 111

Fat 19g

Carbs 18g

Protein 16g

Brownie Muffins

Preparation Time: 10 minutes

Cooking Time: 10 minutes

Servings: 12

Ingredients:

- 1 package Betty Crocker fudge brownie mix
- ¼ cup walnuts, chopped
- 1 egg
- 1/3 cup vegetable oil
- 2 tsp.s water

Directions:

1. Grease 12 muffin molds. Set aside.
2. In a bowl, put all ingredients together.
3. Place the mixture into the prepared muffin molds.
4. Preheat the Air Fryer at 300°F.
5. Arrange the muffin molds in Air Fryer basket and insert in the Air Fryer. Cook for 10 minutes.

6. Place the muffin molds onto a wire rack to cool for about 10 minutes.
7. Carefully, invert the muffins onto the wire rack to completely cool before serving.

Nutrition:

Calories 168

Fat 8.9g

Carbs 20.8g

Protein 2g

Chocolate Mug Cake

Preparation Time: 15 minutes

Cooking Time: 13 minutes

Servings: 1

Ingredients:

- ¼ cup self-rising flour
- 5 tbsp. caster sugar
- 1 tbsp. cocoa powder
- 3 tbsp. coconut oil
- 3 tbsp. whole milk

Directions:

1. In a shallow mug, add all the ingredients and mix until well combined.
2. Preheat the Air Fryer at 392°F.
3. Arrange the mug in Air Fryer basket and insert in the Air Fryer. Cook for 13 minutes.

4. Place the mug onto a wire rack to cool slightly before serving.

Nutrition:

Calories 729

Fat 43.3g

Carbs 88.8g

Protein 5.7g

Grilled Peaches

Preparation Time: 10 minutes

Cooking Time: 10 minutes

Servings: 2

Ingredients:

- 2 peaches, cut into wedges and remove pits
- ¼ cup butter, diced into pieces
- ¼ cup brown sugar
- ¼ cup graham cracker crumbs

Directions:

1. Arrange peach wedges on Air Fryer oven rack and air fry at 350°F for 5 minutes.
2. In a bowl, put the butter, graham cracker crumbs, and brown sugar together.
3. Turn peaches skin side down.
4. Spoon butter mixture over top of peaches and air fry for 5 minutes more.

5. Top with whipped cream and serve.

Nutrition:

Calories 378

Fat 24.4g

Carbs 40.5g

Protein 2.3g

Simple & Delicious Spiced Apples

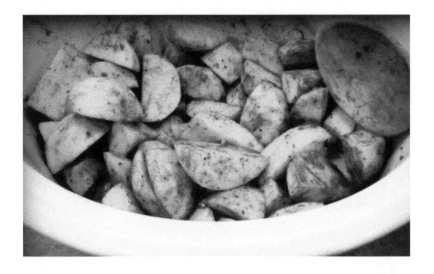

Preparation Time: 10 minutes

Cooking Time: 10 minutes

Servings: 4

Ingredients:

- 4 apples, sliced
- 1 tsp. apple pie spice
- 2 tbsp. sugar

- 2 tbsp. ghee, melted

Directions:

1. Add apple slices into the mixing bowl.
2. Add remaining ingredients on top of apple slices and toss until well coated.
3. Transfer apple slices on Air Fryer oven pan and air fry at 350°F for 10 minutes.
4. Top with ice cream and serve.

Nutrition:

Calories 196

Fat 6.8g

Carbs 37.1g

Protein 0.6g

Tangy Mango Slices

Preparation Time: 10 minutes

Cooking Time: 12 hours

Servings: 6

Ingredients:

- 4 mangoes, peel and cut into ¼-inch slices
- 1/4 cup fresh lemon juice
- 1 tbsp. honey

Directions:

1. In a big bowl, combine together honey and lemon juice and set aside.
2. Add mango slices in lemon-honey mixture and coat well.
3. Arrange mango slices on Air Fryer rack and dehydrate at 135°F for 12 hours.

Nutrition:

Calories 147

Fat 0.9g

Carbs 36.7g

Protein 1.9g

Peanut Butter Cookies

Preparation Time: 10 minutes

Cooking Time: 5 minutes

Servings: 24

Ingredients:

- 1 egg, lightly beaten
- 1 cup of sugar
- 1 cup creamy peanut butter

Directions:

1. In a big bowl, combine sugar, egg, and peanut butter together until well mixed.
2. Spray Air Fryer oven tray with cooking spray.
3. Using ice cream scooper, scoop out cookie onto the tray and flattened them using a fork.
4. Bake cookie at 350°F for 5 minutes.
5. Cook remaining cookie batches using the same temperature.

6. Serve and enjoy.

Nutrition:

Calories 97

Fat 5.6g

Carbs 10.5g

Protein 2.9g

Dried Raspberries

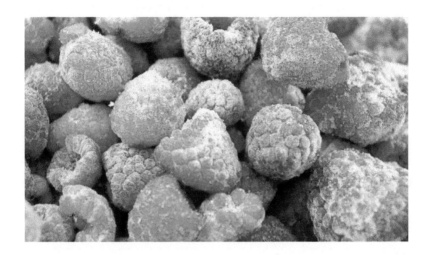

Preparation Time: 10 minutes

Cooking Time: 15 hours

Servings: 4

Ingredients:

- 4 cups raspberries, wash and dry
- 1/4 cup fresh lemon juice

Directions:

1. Add raspberries and lemon juice in a bowl and toss well.
2. Arrange raspberries on Air Fryer oven tray and dehydrate at 135°F for 12-15 hours.
3. Store in an air-tight container.

Nutrition:

Calories 68

Fat 0.9g

Carbs 15g

Protein 1.6g

Sweet Peach Wedges

Preparation Time: 10 minutes

Cooking Time: 8 hours

Servings: 4

Ingredients:

- 3 peaches, cut and remove pits and sliced
- 1/2 cup fresh lemon juice

Directions:

1. Add lemon juice and peach slices into the bowl and toss well.
2. Arrange peach slices on Air Fryer oven rack and dehydrate at 135°F for 6-8 hours.
3. Serve and enjoy.

Nutrition:

Calories 52

Fat 0.5g

Carbs 11.1g

Protein 1.3g

Air Fryer Oreo Cookies

Preparation Time: 5 minutes

Cooking Time: 5 minutes

Servings: 9

Ingredients:

- Pancake Mix: ½ cup
- Water: ½ cup
- Cooking spray
- Chocolate sandwich cookies: 9 (e.g. Oreo)
- Confectioners' sugar: 1 tbsp., or to taste

Directions:

1. Blend the pancake mixture with the water until well mixed.
2. Line the parchment paper on the basket of an Air Fryer. Spray nonstick cooking spray on parchment paper. Dip each cookie into the mixture of the

pancake and place it in the basket. Make sure they do not touch; if possible, cook in batches.

3. The Air Fryer is preheated to 400°F. Add basket and cook for 4 to 5 minutes; flip until golden brown, 2 to 3 more minutes. Sprinkle the sugar over the cookies and serve.

Nutrition:

Calories 77

Fat 2.1g

Carbs 13.7g

Protein 1.2g

Air Fried Butter Cake

Preparation Time: 10 minutes

Cooking Time: 15 minutes

Servings: 4

Ingredients:

- 7 Tbsp. of butter, at ambient temperature
- White sugar: ¼ cup plus 2 tbsp.
- All-purpose flour: 1 ⅔ cups
- Salt: 1 pinch or to taste
- Milk: 6 tbsp.

Directions:

1. Preheat an Air Fryer to 350°F. Spray the cooking spray on a tiny fluted tube pan.
2. Take a large bowl and add ¼ cup butter and 2 tbsp. of sugar in it.
3. Take an electric mixer to beat the sugar and butter until smooth and fluffy. Stir in salt and flour. Stir in

the milk and thoroughly combine batter. Move batter to the prepared saucepan; use a spoon back to level the surface.

4. Place the pan inside the basket of the Air Fryer. Set the timer within 15 minutes. Bake the batter until a toothpick comes out clean when inserted into the cake.

5. Turn the cake out of the saucepan and allow it to cool for about five minutes.

Nutrition:

Calories 470

Fat 22.4g

Carbs 59.7g

Protein 7.9g

Air Fryer S'mores

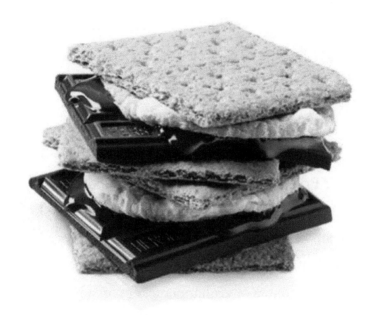

Preparation Time: 5 minutes

Cooking Time: 3 minutes

Servings: 4

Ingredients:

- Four graham crackers (each half split to make 2 squares, for a total of 8 squares)
- 8 Squares of Hershey's chocolate bar, broken into squares
- 4 Marshmallows

Directions:

1. Air Fryers use hot air for cooking food. Marshmallows are light and fluffy, and this should keep the marshmallows from flying around the basket if you follow these steps.
2. Put 4 squares of graham crackers on a basket of the Air Fryer.
3. Place 2 squares of chocolate bars on each cracker.
4. Place back the basket in the Air Fryer and fry on air at 390°F for 1 minute. It is barely long enough for the chocolate to melt. Remove basket from Air Fryer.
5. Top with a marshmallow over each cracker. Throw the marshmallow down a little bit into the melted chocolate. This will help to make the marshmallow stay over the chocolate.
6. Put back the basket in the Air Fryer and fry at 390°F for 2 minutes. (The marshmallows should be puffed up and browned at the tops.)

7. Using tongs to carefully remove each cracker from the basket of the Air Fryer and place it on a platter. Top each marshmallow with another square of graham crackers. Enjoy it right away!

Nutrition:

Calories 200

Fat 3.1g

Carbs 15.7g

Protein 2.6g

Air Fryer chocolate cake

Preparation Time: 6 minutes

Cooking time: 35 minutes

Serving: 9

Ingredients:

- ½cups hot water
- 1 tsp. Vanilla
- ¼cups olive oil
- ½cups almond milk
- 1 egg
- ½ tsp. Salt
- ¾ tsp. Baking soda
- ¾ tsp. Baking powder
- ½cups unsweetened cocoa powder
- 2 cups almond flour
- 1 cup brown sugar

Directions:

1. Preheat your Air Fryer oven to 356°F.
2. Stir all dry ingredients together and then stir in wet ingredients.
3. Add hot water last. The batter should be thin.
4. Pour cake batter into a pan that fits into the fryer.
5. Bake for 35 minutes.

Nutrition:

Calories 378

Fat 9g

Carbs 5g

Protein 4g

Banana Brownies

Preparation Time: 4 minutes

Cooking time: 25 minutes

Servings: 12

Ingredients:

- 1/3 cup almond flour
- tsp. Baking powder
- ½ tsp. Baking soda
- ½ tsp. Salt
- 1 over-ripe banana
- 2 large eggs
- ½ tsp. Stevia powder
- ¼ cup coconut oil
- 1 tbsp. Vinegar
- 1/3 cup cocoa powder

Directions:

1. Preheat the Air Fryer oven for 5 minutes at 350°F.
2. Combine all the listed ingredients in a food processor and pulse until well-combined.
3. Pour into a baking dish that fits in the air fryer.
4. Place in the basket, then cook for 25 minutes, then if a toothpick inserted in the middle comes out clean, take out and let it cool down.

Nutrition:

Calories 75

Fat 6.5g

Carbs 2g

Protein 1.7g

Air fried biscuit donuts

Preparation Time: 7 minutes

Cooking time: 5 minutes

Serving: 8

Ingredients:

- Pinch of allspice
- tbsp. Dark brown sugar
- 1 tsp. Cinnamon
- 1/3cups granulated sweetener
- tbsp. Melted coconut oil
- 1 can of biscuits

Directions:

1. Mix allspice, sugar, sweetener, and cinnamon.
2. Take out biscuits from can and with a circle cookie cutter, cut holes from centers, and place into the Air Fryer.

3. Cook 5 minutes at 350°F
4. As batches are cooked, use a brush to coat with melted coconut oil and dip each into sugar mixture. Serve warm!

Nutrition:

Calories 209

Fat 4g,

Carbs 3g,

Protein 0g

Chocolate soufflé

Preparation Time: 7 minutes

Cooking time: 12 minutes

Serving: 2

Ingredients:

- tbsp. Almond flour
- ½ tsp. Vanilla
- tbsp. Sweetener
- 4 separated eggs
- ¼ cups melted coconut oil
- oz. Of semi-sweet chocolate, chopped

Directions:

1. Preheat the Air Fryer to 330°F.
2. Brush coconut oil and sweetener onto ramekins.
3. Melt coconut oil and chocolate together.
4. Beat egg yolks well, adding vanilla and sweetener.
5. Stir in flour and ensure there are no lumps.

6. Whisk egg whites till they reach peak state and fold them into chocolate mixture.
7. Pour batter into ramekins and place into the Air Fryer oven, then cook for 12 minutes.
8. Serve with powdered sugar dusted on top.

Nutrition:

Calories 238

Fat 6g

Carbs 4g

Protein 1g

Saucy fried bananas

Preparation Time: 7 minutes

Cooking time: 10 minutes

Serving: 2

Ingredients:

- 1 large egg
- ¼ cup cornstarch
- ¼ cup plain breadcrumbs
- bananas, halved crosswise
- Cooking oil
- Chocolate sauce

Directions:

1. Preheat your Air Fryer oven to 350°F.
2. In a small bowl, beat the egg.
3. In another bowl, place the cornstarch.
4. Place the breadcrumbs in a different bowl.

5. Dip the bananas in the cornstarch, then the egg, and then the breadcrumbs.
6. Spray the basket with cooking oil. Place the bananas in the basket and spray them with cooking oil.
7. Cook for 5 minutes.
8. Open the Air Fryer and flip the bananas then cook for an additional 2 minutes.
9. Transfer the bananas to plates.
10. Drizzle the chocolate sauce over the bananas and serve.

Nutrition:

Calories 203

Fat 6g

Protein 3g

Crusty apple hand pies

Preparation Time: 7 minutes

Cooking time: 8 minutes

Servings: 6

Ingredients:

- 15 oz. no-sugar-added apple pie filling
- 1 store-bought crust

Directions:

1. Lay out pie crust and slice into equal-sized squares.
2. Place 2 tbsp. Filling into each square and seal crust with a fork
3. Pour into the oven rack/basket.
4. Set temperature to 390°F and set time to 8 minutes until golden in color.

Nutrition:

Calories 278

Fat 10g,

Carbs 4g

Protein 1g

9 781803 174983